SLOW LEAKS

Missed Opportunities to Encourage Our Engagement in Our Health Care

JESSIE GRUMAN

SLOW LEAKS: Missed Opportunities to Encourage Our
Engagement in Our Health Care

For more information: Health Behavior Media, Center for Advancing
Health, 2000 Florida Avenue, N.W., Suite 210, Washington, D.C.
20009

Published by Health Behavior Media.

Health Behavior Media books are published by
the Center for Advancing Health.

Visit CFAH's website at www.cfah.org

ISBN: 978-0-9815794-1-2

I am indebted to the hundreds of people who have talked with me about their experiences with health care and who have trusted me to transmit their stories in essays that may be helpful to you. I am also deeply grateful to the individuals and foundations that support the work of the Center for Advancing Health to ensure that all of us can act to benefit from our health care.

Find Good Health Care

Make the Most of It

The gap between the demands placed on us by U.S. health care delivery and the ability of individuals — even the most informed and engaged among us — to meet those demands undermines the quality of our care, escalates its cost and diminishes its positive impact on our health.

While advances in medical knowledge have been responsible for steady increases in the length and quality of Americans' lives, the potential of health care to improve individual and population health increasingly depends on us. We must choose the doctors, take the pills, lose the weight, get the tests and show up at the right place at the right time to get the right care.

The stakes of our engagement for us and the nation have never been higher. There is evidence that the more engaged we are in our care, the better we do. And conversely, our lack of involvement contributes to preventable illness, complications and sometimes death. It wastes precious health care resources and can negatively affect the health of those of us who are unable to participate effectively in our care.

What does it take for us and our families to find good care and make the most of it? And what can be done to help those who lack the skills, resources or capacities, or who are already ill, compensate for their inability to do so?

The essays in this collection* identify some of the key challenges posed to most of us by health care as it is currently delivered in many settings. None of these challenges is monumental, but each one contributes to the steady erosion in quality of care and to a waste of resources. Each essay identifies a "slow leak" that saps value from the services and technologies we receive and suggests solutions that would benefit us and those who work with us to improve our health.

*The essays in this collection were originally published on the Prepared Patient Blog from January 2011 through May 2012.[1]

Engagement Does Not Mean Compliance

Twenty percent of people who leave their doctors' offices with a new prescription don't fill it.[1] Up to half of those who do fill their prescriptions don't take the drugs as recommended.[2,3] These individuals are considered non-compliant. But does that mean they are not engaged in their health care? "Engagement" and "compliance" are not synonyms.

I am compliant if I do what my doctor tells me to do.

I am engaged when I actively participate in the process of solving my health problems. A new prescription is an element in that process. If I am engaged in my care, I might want to learn about this medication, such as: *What can it do and not do to ease my pain or slow the progress of my disease? What side effects might it produce and what should I do about them? How long will it take to work? When should I take it and how? How much does it cost? What will happen if I don't take it?*

I might want to consider the barriers to taking it and weigh the risks and benefits of alternatives. Could I instead make changes in my physical activity level or diet, try a dietary supplement, or watchfully wait to see if the symptoms subside?

If my clinician has done more than just hand me the prescription — if she has, for example, raised these questions and discussed these concerns with me, I probably won't have a prescription in my hand if I don't intend to fill it.

But I can be engaged in my health care even if I don't have that conversation with my provider. I can ponder each of these questions with family and friends. I can search the library and Google for answers. I can consult online with others who have taken that medication. And sure, I'll accept the prescription in case I decide to fill it. But I make no guarantee.

The rhetoric of engagement is attractive to all of us: patients, providers, hospitals, employers and health plans. That rhetoric says that patients have "choices" about our health care, that we are "empowered" to participate actively in our health care. And of course, that it's time we "take responsibility" for our health.

Many who speak about the need for us to engage in our health care confuse compliance with engagement. They assume that the only rational choice we can make is to behave consistently with our clinicians' directives, whether that means filling a prescription, losing weight or undergoing surgery.

But this is not how many of us hear these messages. The rhetoric says we have choices? We hear, "You have the power to choose which doctor to consult and which advice you will follow." It says we are empowered to find good health solutions? We hear, "Your Web searches and new friends online can help you figure out what to do as well as your doctor can." The rhetoric says we are responsible for our health and health care? We hear, "You are on your own." What we hear is reinforced by reality: a paucity of clinicians who encourage and welcome our participation in our care and office visits that rarely allow time for in-depth conversations.

Saying "engagement" when meaning "compliance" reinforces the belief that we are the only ones who must change our behavior. Doing so misrepresents the magnitude of shifts in attitude, expectations and effort that are required for all health care stakeholders to ensure that we have adequate knowledge and support to make well-informed decisions. And it fails to recognize that our behaviors are powerfully shaped by many contingencies: money, culture, time, illness status and personal preference. Being engaged in our health and care does not mean following our clinicians' instructions to the letter. Rather, it means being able to accurately weigh the benefits and risks of taking a new medication, stopping smoking or getting a PSA test in the context of the many other demands and opportunities that influence our pursuit of lives that are free of suffering for ourselves and those we love.

Find Good Health Care

The Rocky Adolescence of Public Reporting on Health Care Quality

Our ailing economy has boosted the number of people who are unemployed, without health insurance or with minimal coverage.[1-3] The popularity of high-deductible health plans is soaring as employers and individuals look for affordable insurance. Twenty-nine percent of personal bankruptcies are said to be caused by medical bills.[4] Many of us now choose health care services and providers based on cost, trying to stay within tight budgets.

The American people, long protected from the price of health care by insurance, are now forced to act as consumers. This situation is a free marketer's dream. According to this model, we will rationally calculate the price and quality trade-offs of each doctor visit, procedure, test and drug. We will stop overusing services. We will demand better care. And the result will be reduced health care costs for the nation while the quality of care and the health of individuals will remain the same, if not improve.

There's nothing like a good theory.

But the theory can be tested only if a) it's easy to find publicly reported, relevant quality information about the services we need, matched with what we would pay out of pocket; and b) we use that information as the basis of our health care decisions. Neither of these conditions can be met today.

A systematic review of evidence titled "Public release of performance data in changing the behavior of healthcare consumers, professionals or organizations" reiterates what previous reviews on this topic have found: There is little evidence that public reporting produces meaningful, long-term changes in individuals' choices about their care.[5-7] This review examined four studies that consisted of 35,000 potential patients and 1,560 hospitals. It found that the public reporting of performance data had no effect on people's choice of health plans. In one of the studies, reporting mortality and complication data on two specific surgeries had a small impact on people's choices about where to have those surgeries performed for two months following the release of the information.

What kind of information do public reporting advocates believe will shape our decisions about care? Composite measures of hospital safety? Patient satisfaction ratings based on the Consumer Assessment of Healthcare Providers and Systems (CAHPS)? Report cards on specific outcomes of specific surgeries? With the possible exception of CAHPS, currently available quality information seems based on small elements of clinical care that can be measured with minimal burden. This may be useful for clinicians and administrators, but not for us patients.

Focus groups consistently find that people want to know answers to questions such as: Who can I trust to tell me if I really need back surgery? Where should I go to get a hip replacement that will allow me to walk well again? Who can really help me get my diabetes under control? Information that answers our questions and is presented so we can make sense of what is available where and when we need it from a trustworthy source does not exist.[8] Cost information for specific services, tests and procedures is almost impossible to find and is rarely matched with corresponding quality information.[9]

It's early in the performance measurement business. Advances in computer technology have only recently made it possible to collect quality information on a broad scale. Paul Shekelle, M.D., Ph.D., of RAND noted that after public reporting (in combination with incentives to change clinician and institutional behavior) produced a few small victories (such as an increase in the use of beta blockers after a heart attack), unintended consequences of both measurement and reporting sometimes emerged.[10,11] Shekelle adds, "Be careful what you measure and report, since this action will distort the system, and you want to make sure you are distorting it for the good!"

Meanwhile, buckets of money pour into quality measurement and improvement. Eventually this field will mature, probably in lock step with the lumbering implementation of electronic health records.[12] But without meaningful quality indicators and timely reporting along dimensions that can really improve care and that patients care about, maturity will merely produce new wrinkles in lieu of wisdom.

The lack of good, relevant quality and price information to help us make decisions is only one barrier, however. Our orientation toward being knowledgeable, active participants in our care is also immature. We have no tradition of exercising critical judgment about our health care. We don't believe that its technical quality varies.[13] Many of us believe that the higher the cost, the better the care. Most of us have little understanding of how health care is organized or how our insurance works. We don't know whether our physician is part of a practice, a clinic, a hospital or an accountable care organization and why that matters. Our connection is with our doctor — that's the level at which we understand and care about quality. Further, most of us don't know how to ferret out the price of an individual service, procedure or test even if we need that information.

So this is where we are today: a juvenile collection of performance measurement and public reporting initiatives aimed at influencing a public that is largely unprepared (uninformed, unwilling and often unable) to do the currently difficult work of finding information that can help us make good health care choices.

I have few illusions that the growth in the cost of health care will be slowed through our efforts, even if most of us make well-informed decisions based on price/quality trade-offs. Shoshanna Sofaer, Dr.P.H., of CUNY reminds me that the targets of public reporting choices are not the big budget items driving health care expenditures. After all, 5 percent of the population accounts for 49 percent of health care expenses.[14,15] The cost-saving efforts of garden-variety patients will always only nibble around the edges. Few of us will disaggregate the costly treatment of a brain tumor, for example, into price and quality bits: this neurologist, the neurosurgeon who will do the operation for half the price of the other, an oncologist in the neighboring town, a cheaper radiologist down the street. We have other things to worry about at that point.

Now, however, the need to make good decisions about our care in the absence of relevant price and quality information has the potential to erode our individual health. There is already evidence that our decisions to delay needed care and titrate our drugs because we can't afford them are not informed or smart ones: We are just sicker when we eventually do seek care.[16] Those who are most likely to need price and quality information are likely to already be ill and lack the energy, skills and resources to use the information, even if it were easy to find and understandable.

This will change over time: Quality measurement will mature and eventually will produce information that is relevant, interesting and useful to us. Our personal mastery of health information online and the critical attitude we are acquiring will continue to grow, prompted by the economic necessity to be informed and involved.[17]

In the meantime, public reporting on health care quality is experiencing a rocky adolescence. The assumptions behind the theory that people's informed, rational choices of better quality, lower-cost care will shape the market and "bend the cost curve" have yet to be met. The immature status of public reporting on health care metrics, combined with our general passivity, means most of us still operate as semi-educated guessers, making semi-OK, sometimes semi-disastrous decisions based on the advice of our doctors, convenience, familiarity, a little Google searching and the suggestions of friends.

What Must We Know About What Our Doctors Know?

> "The most important thing I learned was that different doctors know different things: I need to ask my internist different questions than I do my oncologist."

This was not some sweet ingénue recounting the early lessons she learned from a recent encounter with health care. Nope. It was a 62-year-old woman whose husband has been struggling with multiple myeloma for the last eight years and who herself has chronic back pain, high blood pressure and high cholesterol and was at the time well into treatment for breast cancer.

Part of me says, "Ahem. Have you been paying attention here?" and another part says, "Well, of course! How were you supposed to know this? Have any of your physicians ever described their scope of expertise or practice to you?"

I can see clinicians rolling their eyes at the very thought of having such a discussion with every patient. And I can imagine some of us on the receiving end thinking that, when these topics are raised by a clinician, they are little more than disclaimers, an avoidance of accountability and liability.

But all of us — particularly those who receive care from more than one doctor — need to have a rudimentary idea of what each clinician we consult knows and does. Why is this clinician referring me to someone else? How will she communicate with that clinician going forward? How and about what does she hope I will communicate with her in the future?

Why does our clinician need to address these questions?

Because in the absence of real guidance, we will guess. Some of us will make informed guesses and be mostly right. Others of us will leave our primary care provider in the dust and seek care for routine health matters from our specialist, whom we see more frequently and who seems to know us better. Some of us, like my friend above, will ask for help from whichever physician is handy and will call back, regardless of the problem. And some of us will throw up our hands in frustration and head for the local emergency department when we find we can't breathe and don't know which of our doctors to consult about those damn allergies.

These ad hoc solutions are a waste of our time and surely contribute to a poor use of clinician and institutional resources.

Fragmentation of health care and lack of coordination of services are widely recognized as problems.[1,2] Considerable efforts now aim to improve communication among providers when a person leaves the hospital, for example, and great stock is placed in the potential of new patient-centered medical homes to "coordinate" our care (although the parameters of such coordination have yet to be defined).[3,4]

There has been little or no recognition, however, of the fact that we patients and our families and loved ones are the main coordinators of all care: We decide when a threshold of discomfort has been crossed and we need professional help. We decide from whom and in what setting to seek such help. And for the foreseeable future, unfortunately, we choose to share the test results and treatment plans from one of our clinicians with another — or not. And we are doing this without guidance.

What would guidance look like?

Well, it doesn't look like a website. More likely it has clinicians taking these three small steps:

Clearly introducing their expertise, their experience and their role relative to other clinicians caring for us. This needn't be highly technical or take a lot of time, but it does need to differentiate one clinician's role from that of other specialists or primary care providers, anticipating that I and my caregivers may be confused about which problem is best addressed by which doctor. Connie Davis, a geriatric nurse practitioner in British Columbia, says, "When I introduce myself to the patients I serve, I say, 'I'm a geriatric nurse practitioner. Have you ever worked with a nurse practitioner before?' If they haven't, I tell them that I am a nurse with additional training, so I am somewhere between a nurse and a doctor and that I work with older adults to address common health concerns and make sure everything is working as well as possible."

Giving simple but full explanations about referrals: why, to whom, for what, expectations about ongoing care and future communication, both between physicians and between the referring clinician and the patient. Such an explanation lays out a template for us to more easily find the right solution to the current problem. Further, many of us assume that because the receptionist uses a computer, our records are automatically electronically (and magically) transmitted to every physician to whom we are referred. We can't do our part to support inter-physician communication if we believe it is being done for us already.

Saying, "That's not my area of expertise." As someone who is "doctored up" with about 15 physicians treating me right now, I sometimes guess wrong about what any one of them considers within his expertise. I get a little frustrated but am ultimately reassured when one of them responds to my question with "Not my body part," or "You need to talk to your primary care provider about that." A survey by the National Alliance on Mental Illness found that patients and family members are concerned when their doctors don't tell them they lack expertise about a condition: 75 percent of parents of kids with mental illness who were surveyed doubt the ability of their primary care providers to treat their kids effectively.[5,6] It's difficult to establish a "continuous healing relationship," as the Institute of Medicine report Crossing the Quality Chasm encourages, when questions about clinician competencies are not directly addressed.[7]

Don't get me wrong. System-level fixes such as tailored online information, interoperable electronic health records with good patient portals and enhanced primary care will ease some of the redundancy and fill some of the gaps that now by default (and often without our recognition) fall to us to patch together. But at the end of the day, it's my mom deciding whether to call the cardiologist, the neurologist, the geriatrician or 911 about my disabled dad's sudden dizziness. She's the one who coordinates his care.

She needs help from her clinicians to fulfill this responsibility. As do we all.

Semper Paratus: Our Decisions About Emergency Care

Nora misjudged the height of the stair outside the restaurant, stepped down too hard, jammed her knee and tore her meniscus. Not that we knew this at the time. All we knew then was that she was howling from the pain.

There we were on a dark, empty, wet street in lower Manhattan, not a cab in sight, with a wailing, immobile woman. What to do? Call 911? Find a cab to take her home and contact her primary care doctor for advice? Take her home, put ice on her knee, feed her Advil and call her doctor in the morning?

Sometimes it is clear that the only response to a health crisis is to call 911 and head for the emergency department (ED). But in this case — and in so many others we encounter with our kids, our parents, our co-workers and on the street — while the demand for some action is urgent, the course of action is less obvious.

The question "which action?" has become more complicated of late because:

- In some communities, there are alternatives to an ambulance or a drive to the nearest ED, such as urgent care centers.[1]

- Disincentives exist for going the route of the ED. In many cash-strapped municipalities, we are charged for the cost of an ambulance ride. Or we risk not having our ED visit covered by insurance if we make the wrong decision or fail to notify our health plan in a timely manner. Or we don't have insurance and ED care is expensive.[2,3]

- Some of us have a number of clinicians who could guide us about ED versus self care on any urgent health matter, plus our health plan may have a nurse advice line that could do the same. Which among them to call? How long will it take to get an answer in the middle of a busy workday or a late night?

- Many of us have no primary care clinician to call.[4]

What hasn't changed is that sense of panic. We don't know enough to judge how serious the situation is. We feel tremendous pressure to do something to resolve the pain and don't know how to do it ourselves, but we don't want to be responsible for underestimating the problem and causing additional harm.

Efforts to help us problem-solve quickly about urgent health events have been going on for a while. For example, The *Healthwise® Handbook*, distributed to more than 33 million people since 1975, walks readers efficiently through such decisions. The handbook information is available to everyone for free on WebMD and HolaDoctor at http://www.healthwise.org/Questions.aspx.[5] The American College of Emergency Physicians has a good list posted on its site and elsewhere of general indicators for when to go to the ED.[6,7] Other large health sites provide varied levels of advice about responding to specific health emergencies. But finding the right guidance fast depends on our ability to know about a good source for relevant information, to locate that source — the book or the search term or nurse-line number — then to read and understand how it applies to the urgent situation at the moment.

Such efforts seem haphazard in light of two facts: First, that Americans made 136.1 million visits to the ED in 2008, and second, that a good number of these visits were not for urgent conditions.[8,9] It's true that the ED is the only place that some of us can get health care, and considerable attention is directed toward reducing visits by frequent users.[10,11] But none of us is immune to making the wrong call. Our decisions about where to seek care for a health crisis are made largely in the absence of knowledge or expert advice, wasting our time and money as well as that of professionals and institutions.[12,13]

Health crises are common in the population, but rare among individuals. Regardless of our experience, when one happens to us, to a family member or a co-worker or in front of us on the Little League field, we know we must act. Right now, despite all the options and disincentives for doing so, the default action for most of us is calling 911 or going to the ED. We would benefit from a little help here.

So come on, those of you who have a stake in making health care more patient-centered! This is an easy win.

If you are a primary care clinician in a practice or a medical home, tell your patients how you and your staff handle emergencies both during the day and after hours.[14] Who should they call? What can they expect? Post this information, send it to them, remind them about it when you see them.

If you are an employer, make sure your employees know what services you have purchased for them as part of their insurance benefit to help them respond to an emergency. Show them where this information is located on the premium information website or in the handbook; remind them about that nurse advice line.

If you work for a health plan, communicate directly, clearly and consistently with beneficiaries about their specific benefit: What must they do to ensure care is covered? Where on the plan website is there information that could help in making decisions about emergency care?

If you work on patient-centered care for the government, form a partnership across agencies and with private industry to gather the lessons from the 911 experience to inform the development and promotion of a self-triage emergency app for smartphones. Create something that every one of us could use when a health condition turns serious or an accident occurs — something that provides guidance to distinguish ED-level emergencies from "put ice on it and take some ibuprofen." By the time you do this, smartphones should be in the hands of most Americans.[15]

Ideally, care that is patient-centered is organized to enable us to act to optimally benefit from the knowledge, services and technologies available to us. Each of these strategies would help us do so.

So what happened to Nora? She figured that since she wasn't bleeding and probably didn't break any bones, going home and getting advice from her primary care physician might save her a cold night on a hard chair in the local ED. She's hobbling but healing.

Slow Leaks: Missed Opportunities to Encourage Our Engagement in Our Health Care

Dicker With Your Doc? Not So Fast

"How to Haggle With Your Doctor" was the title of a Business section column in *The New York Times* a while ago.[1] This is one of many similar directives to the public in magazines and on TV and websites urging us to lower the high price of our health care by going mano a mano with our physicians about the price of tests they recommend and the drugs they prescribe.[2-4] Such articles provide simple, common-sense recommendations about how to respond to the urgency many of us — insured or uninsured — feel to reduce our health care expenses.

With unemployment at 9.4 percent and more than 50 million Americans lacking any or adequate health insurance as I write this in January 2011, I understand the impulse of editors to assign this story. Plus, "of all the providers of medical care, physicians are most important in determining how much will be spent," notes Arnold Relman in the *New York Review of Books*, since they make all the allocation decisions that "call on the facilities and services of all the other providers of care — hospitals, imaging centers, diagnostic laboratories, manufacturers of drugs and equipment."[5] The prices charged by these institutions vary widely, and therein lies the opportunity to find some savings.

But, coming off a wave of big-buck, out-of-pocket spending related to my recent diagnosis of stomach cancer, I am acutely aware that haggling with my doctor about the costs of my care is neither simple nor a matter of common sense. Rather, it is a matter of 1) understanding in detail both the opportunities and limitations related to my health insurance; 2) being persistent in seeking information, since price lists are often difficult to track down and comparisons of quality (accuracy) of laboratories and testing facilities are nonexistent; 3) using available information and my judgment to weigh options; 4) being willing to risk the rejection of my request by my provider and perhaps antagonize her; and 5) overcoming my pride and asking to be treated well while paying less than everyone else.

The fact that health care is not a real "market" for patients is old news, although perhaps not to the writers of these articles who blithely recommend that we set off to haggle our way to cheaper care. And it is irrelevant news to the vast majority of the public for whom discussing cost with their doctor is anathema. Many people would not consider doing so; first, because they may not know that the prices of drugs and tests vary so much by provider or source; second, because they may feel uncomfortable mentioning money concerns; and third, because Americans have long held the view that more expensive care is better care, and in seeking to pay less, one may be tacitly agreeing to accept less effective care.[6]

Objectively, none of these factors should influence a person's ability to ask straightforwardly: "I wonder if there is a way you could help me reduce the price of my care?" But our relationship with our providers is rarely objective. We come to them when we are sick and vulnerable. We put our lives in their hands. We trust them to do the best for us. And we value deeply their efforts. Haggle about the price of this commitment? Many of us will not, even if the alternatives are bankruptcy or going without care.

So what should we make of this rash of recommendations to enlist our providers in reducing the price of care?

I, for one, want to know whether doctors and other providers can easily find the information they need so that if we must ask for help to pay less, they are able to respond with useful strategies and without hostility. All health plans remind doctors of policies that aim to constrain costs by providing incentives to those who deliver care that is evidence-based, for example, or dictating the priorities of drugs prescribed for certain treatments.[7-8] But our requests are not policy-based. They relate to the use of specific facilities, drugs and tests. Other than providers in federally qualified health centers, many of whom have well-honed skills in squeezing the most care from each dollar, most providers are largely unfamiliar with the prices of the services and technologies they recommend.

Will this advice to ask for a break on the price of care exert demand that results in more transparency about cost and quality? Perhaps, but only if many more people cast off their traditional passivity with regard to their care, overcome their reluctance to discuss money, and invest the time required to track down the elusive price and quality information that is required.

The frequency of the recommendation to haggle with one's doctor may reassure the public that discussing the price of care will apply pressure to meaningfully reduce what we pay. But saying "This drug/that test is too expensive for me. Can you do me a favor and spend time with me to find lower price solutions without compromising quality?" is not an approach that will lead to a widespread and enduring solution.

While we are waiting for the enactment of federal and state policies that would ensure that each of us can afford the care we need, what private policies and public regulations about transparency and price would help us out here? What would ensure that those of us who are willing to take on the task of trying to cut a better deal for our care with our providers have the information and guidance to do so?

Are Patient Navigators Necessary or Just Nice?

Each of the four times I have received a cancer-related diagnosis, I felt like I had been drop-kicked into a foreign country: I didn't know the language, I didn't understand the culture, I didn't have a map, and I desperately wanted to find my way home.

Over the years I have listened to hundreds of people describe the same experience following the diagnosis of a serious illness. As the number of physicians, diagnostic test sites and treatment options have grown and the lack of seamless, coordinated care persists, the majority of patients and their loved ones struggle to find the right care and make good use of it. [1]

It makes sense, then, to add to the collection of health professionals one meets on this particular journey a "navigator" who can remove barriers to care and help fill gaps in knowledge and skills that anxious patients and their loved ones encounter during this stressful time.

Indeed, it has made so much sense to so many people working in health care that there is now a thriving movement to train and employ patient navigators in a variety of settings. [2]

To quote Butch Cassidy, "Who are those guys anyway?"

What are patient navigators?

In 1990, Harold P. Freeman, M.D., pioneered the first patient navigator program at Harlem Hospital to help shorten the time between the diagnosis of cancer and beginning treatment. [3] The navigators were former cancer patients, and the program was successful in achieving this aim. [4] Since then, the navigator concept has exploded. You now can find patient navigators deployed to help people make their way through treatment for breast cancer, cancer in general, various tests, and for a multitude of chronic conditions and populations (at-risk women, older people, etc.).[5-9]

And what do they do? The descriptions of navigators' activities include greeting and concierge-type interactions at hospitals, coordinating appointments, accompanying patients to appointments and tests, explaining tests and treatments, counseling for psychosocial distress, and referring to community services.[10-12]

Training to become a navigator corresponds with these diverse activities. Some patient navigator programs are staffed solely by professionals with extra training: medical social workers or nurses.[13] Others require no background in health, only some training in "navigating," which ranges from learning health content over the course of two hours, two days or two months.[14,15] Some patient navigators are volunteers, some earn minimum wage and some are paid as professionals. There are some fledgling efforts to certify patient navigators, but the recognition of that certification appears to be mostly local.

How is the effectiveness of patient navigator programs measured? It is difficult to find a description of the expected impact of navigator programs and thus little information is available about whether and how programs and hospitals evaluate whether they are fulfilling their stated functions. There are only a few published articles on this topic.[16,17] No single list of expected outcomes of patient navigation or metrics to account for them appears to be widely used.

Who pays for patient navigators? Pharmaceutical companies have invested heavily, as have some individual philanthropists.[18] The federal government supports a number of research programs to develop and test models for patient navigators. Navigators play a role in many of the National Cancer Institute Community Cancer Centers and are sponsored by many local units of the American Cancer Society.

And how widespread is patient navigation? Hard to tell. The media have taken a shine to the idea. And it has produced many employment opportunities: Enter "patient navigators" on any job website search

Slow Leaks: Missed Opportunities to Encourage Our Engagement in Our Health Care

field. You'll be amazed.

What's wrong with this picture? Well, aside from concerns about quality control, the possibility of patients receiving misleading information, and program instability due to a lack of a sustainable revenue model, I suppose this general "let a thousand flowers bloom" approach is OK. It sure makes for a lot of nice ancillary support for some patients in some places.

But this is not good enough. Our lack of sufficient skills and knowledge about how to find the right care and make good use of it causes real problems for many of us. We vary in our experience with illness and health literacy, but none of us is prepared to confront the complex information-and-service-seeking requirements of health care today, especially when we are frightened and ill. The consequences of our lack of preparation are delays, poor decisions about providers and treatment, sporadic follow-through and low adherence to recommended tests and treatment. This harms us, contributes to poor outcomes and wastes resources: ours, our employers' and our government's.

These are problems that are necessary to solve as part of the effort to improve the quality and effectiveness of our care. They are not merely nice to address with optional auxiliary services.

The current haphazard approach to meeting these needs adds to the fragmentation of our care and deepens our confusion about the roles and responsibilities of our care providers. It pushes technical responsibilities to lower-paid non-professionals who lack accountability for outcomes. The informal position of patient navigation within quality measurement and improvement programs allows hospitals to claim they address critical care coordination concerns while abdicating responsibility for them.

In the late '90s, I met with the president of a major disability insurer to ask her if she would be willing to implement a patient-navigator-type program for people with chronic diseases. She said, "Sure. But to do this, I need a scope of work. I need to know who to hire, what skills they have, what training they need and how their qualifications are certified. I need to know what outcomes I can expect with what level of effort over what time. Give me this information and if it will help beneficiaries without breaking the bank, I'll pay for it."

Can this be done for patient navigators? Agreed-upon aims, evidence about effectiveness, description of required skills, scope of work and well-defined metrics for assessment are necessary so that — in this time of evidence-based health care — programs can be implemented that ensure we have the guidance and support we need to make the best possible use of the services and treatments available to us.

If this information is not available, what will it take to produce it? And if it doesn't exist, or if there is no commitment to producing it, should patient navigation just continue to meander along?

Giving patient navigation a credible, reliable place in health care delivery would mean that some of what currently goes on under the rubric of patient navigation may be spun off and delegated to other providers: health coaching, case management, social work, patient advocacy, care coordination. All of these job titles represent attempts to fill the gaps that patients experience in their care. They, too, should be held to standards of safety and effectiveness.

We need reliable, competent help to find our way through complex health care practices and treatments if we are to fully benefit from the care available to us.

Want to make a real contribution to patient-centered care? Invest in developing evidence-based, reliably-delivered patient navigation that will help us do so.

Are We All Ready for Do-It-Yourself Health Care?

The outsourcing of work by businesses to the cheapest available workers has received a lot of attention in recent years. It has largely escaped notice, however, that the new labor force isn't necessarily located in Southeast Asia but is often found here at home and is virtually free. It is us, using our laptops and smartphones to perform more and more functions once carried out by knowledgeable salespeople and service reps.

This was particularly salient to me this week as I spent an hour online browsing, comparing prices, reading customer reviews, and filling out the required billing and shipping information to get a great deal on a new lamp. An airline would charge me 99 cents to talk to a person but provides information for free online. Calls to Amtrak to make train reservations are routinely answered with a message that the wait to talk to an agent is 30 minutes, but that I can book travel myself — plus get better deals — if I do it online. My bank has a small staff, limited hours, and it charges extra for paper checks and mailed hard copy statements...but its website is welcoming and useful, even at 3 a.m.

Many of us don't really mind taking on these additional responsibilities. We are pleased with the convenience of doing these tasks ourselves. We like the mastery we gain by looking at all the options and choosing the best one for us. And we don't even seem to mind the shared accountability these do-it-yourself approaches impose: When we mess up, it's our own fault.

But as online applications make it easier to find better, more convenient deals on goods and services, the old way of doing business has become more expensive and less available: The incentives are aligned to make our patronage online the best and, increasingly, the only choice.

There is considerable cyber-optimism about the cost-cutting potential of health applications — electronic health records, secure messaging with clinicians and weight loss programs.[1,2] Even blood pressure and diabetes monitoring can be designed to capitalize on the efficiency and personalization offered online.

But the stream of surveys and studies documenting just who among us does not — for various reasons — make use of existing online applications for health-related purposes should give pause to patient advocates, health professionals and health policy makers.[3]

Why?

The migration of service from in-person to online comes with the assumption by the sponsor that if we can explore, investigate, compare, communicate and purchase online, we will.

The article "The Digital Divide in Adoption and Use of a Personal Health Record" in the *Archives of Internal Medicine* suggests otherwise.[4] Cyrus Yamin and his colleagues studied a large population with uniform access to an online personal health record (PHR) through which they could view their medication lists, laboratory results, appointment information and could communicate electronically with their clinicians' practice. Of 75,056 people, only 43 percent had made any use of this service, and half of those who did logged in only once. Blacks and Hispanics were half as likely as whites to make use of the PHR. Interestingly, race and ethnicity was far less strongly associated with intensity of use among all those who did register.

It is easy to be lulled into believing that the lack of Internet use is a temporary problem that will be soon solved by the access afforded by the growing popularity of smartphones. Yamin's research suggests that access to the Internet is only one barrier for those of us who lack literacy and search skills, experience, cultural orientation, confidence or cognitive capacity (because we are ill or frightened or frail) to use the online information and applications upon which we increasingly must depend — or face expensive consequences. Because today:

We are responsible for carrying out our own treatments. Advances in drugs and technology make it possible for us to administer complex treatments ourselves. For example, we return home from the hospital quicker but sicker and have become, along with our families, responsible for our drug, dietary, medication and rehabilitation regimens. We operate in-home medical devices for infusions, oxygen, drains, dialysis and feeding. We take multiple medications that require constant monitoring and dietary and physical activity modification. We often struggle to do these things competently.[5] Information, guidance and applications are available online that can help us organize, track and administer treatments to ourselves and our loved ones and help us know when and who to call for help when our efforts fall short.

Certain information is available only online. Comparative quality ratings for nursing homes, hospitals and doctors are available only online. Medicare Part D was designed for online use by older Americans (or their children).[6] It is far easier to compare and find the best deal for individual health insurance policies online.[7] Decision support tools for various treatments are available in print only sporadically and cannot be tailored to one's specific condition as they can be online.[8]

Interactions about our health care are increasingly conducted online. The drive to increase the meaningful use of personal health records consigns administrative functions such as scheduling, updating or correcting our medical and insurance histories to us, the no-cost workforce, just as it has for Amtrak and my bank (some advocates will sigh, "Dream on..." here).[9] As the *Archives* article demonstrates, the intuitive appeal to "do it ourselves" is far from universal.

Let's not kid ourselves. Just because we go online doesn't mean we are using that access for meaningful health-related purposes. Just because important, useful applications exist doesn't mean we seek or find them. And just because we find them doesn't mean we act on the information they provide.

But even today, to obtain the full benefit of health information and health care services, we are required to make use of online applications, which in turn means that a substantial percentage of us must rapidly acquire health literacy skills, rudimentary knowledge about our bodies and health care, and some technological sophistication — and that we overthrow a lifetime of habit to transform ourselves from passive to active participants in our care. The consequences of not doing so are expensive in terms of our money, time and health.

Those who are unable or unwilling to respond to incentives and marketing efforts to actively engage with the health tools and information online are losing...again.

Why Can I Get Health Care Only from 9–5, M–F?

Last week, the waiting room of the outpatient cancer clinic looked like an airport lounge without the rolling suitcases. There were about 20 of us cancer survivor-types talking on our smartphones, fiddling with our iPads, reading *The New York Times*. A few of us were sipping delicious boysenberry-flavored contrast fluid in preparation for a scan, but most of us were waiting to meet with our oncologists for follow-up or monitoring visits. All of us were between the ages of 20 and 70 and all of us were dressed for success — or at least for our jobs.

What's wrong with this picture? Why were all of us employed adults spending a busy Wednesday morning waiting to visit our oncologists or get a test when we should have been working?

We were there because the doctors, the labs and the testing services of this cancer center operate only during standard business hours, which is also when we are supposed to be working. And this means that something's gotta give if the growing number of us cancer survivors are going to attend to the ongoing chronic conditions caused by our treatment and be monitored for recurrences. In the meantime, what's gotta give is us and our employers.

Katherine Evans, a four-time cancer survivor who works in the financial services industry in New York City, has a lot of experience with this problem. "I looked at how much time it really takes to do all the scheduling, going to appointments, testing — preventive care and maintenance — and realized that most of it has to be done between 9–5 on a weekday. I estimate that it takes roughly 15–20 percent of my workweek — almost one full day every week! I count myself lucky I have an understanding manager."

Lest we limit this problem to the privileged group of people who have been treated for cancer and who are able to work, consider that in 2007, a full 39 percent of the working-age population — 72 million people in the U.S. — had at least one chronic health condition: asthma, diabetes, heart disease, depression, arthritis, HIV/AIDS. This number continues to grow.[1]

The treatment approach that offers those of us with chronic conditions the best chance of remaining healthy and active is based on the Chronic Care Model, which calls for proactive, planned testing and monitoring with a health care clinician periodically throughout the year, rather than waiting for acute episodes or complications to drive us to care.[2]

Making and keeping appointments during the current usual hours of health care delivery (i.e., 9-to-5, Monday through Friday) has become more challenging for working patients in the past few years for a number of reasons: We are contracting chronic conditions at a younger age; the Baby Boom generation is aging; economic conditions mean many of us must continue to work long past the age of 65.

Further, because of advances in early detection, treatment and symptom management, many of us with serious chronic conditions are able to remain in the workforce, contributing to the support of our families and our communities and paying for our health insurance.

These shifts in demographics, technology and best practices come together in a perfect storm of need for workers with chronic conditions to have access to non-urgent health care outside the 9-to-5 weekday window.

There has been some recognition of this need: Federally Qualified Health Centers and free clinics are among the leaders in making all kinds of care available after working hours and on weekends, as have Kaiser Permanente and some other health systems.[3] Similarly, some diagnostic facilities and laboratories are open in the early morning and evening. Free-standing urgent care centers have extended hours, are open 365 days a year and increasingly offer routine lab services — sometimes even mammograms.

Celeste Lee, an administrator at the University of Michigan, who has lived with end-stage renal disease for 30 years, notes: "Dialysis units have increased the number of shifts and options for start times, making it easier to fit in a full-time job. On the other hand, they do not make it easy to get on the shift you need. Sometimes those are already taken up by others who are not working."

But clinicians have been slow to routinely extend their hours for working patients. Michael Millenson, in a *Kaiser Health News* blog discussing the safety threats of 9-to-5 hospital professional staff coverage, suggests that this is going to be a heavy lift: Hospitals, like most outpatient settings, "remain the doctor's workshop, dependent upon the goodwill of physicians who admit and care for patients."[4] Further, "telling a neurosurgeon, 'You're working Wednesday through Sunday this week' would rank high on the list of what a friend of mine calls a 'career-limiting event.'"

While I am not talking here about anything as radical as forcing neurosurgeons to operate on Sundays (Heaven forbid!), I am raising the question of how physician practices can best help their patients with chronic conditions get the care they need.

After all, limited hours for ambulatory care delivery means our employers lose. They lose because we are frequently absent. They lose our time and attention when we are at work, because we must schedule appointments and consult with our clinicians by phone during working hours, the only time it is possible to accomplish these tasks. And they lose when the demands of our workplace are such that keeping our job takes precedence over keeping healthy.

And patients lose, too. We are distracted by hours spent trying to unobtrusively schedule our appointments, coordinate our care and get our test results sent to the right clinicians. Our frequent health care visits during working hours mean we are absent for at least half a day multiple times during the year. Sometimes we use our carefully hoarded sick leave.[5] Sometimes we make up the work after hours. Attending to health care during working hours adds significantly to the price we pay for our care: Those of us who are self-employed or are hourly workers simply don't get paid for this time, which means that a fair number of us don't have the option to sit in that waiting room at all.

Helen Darling, president and CEO of the National Business Group on Health, says, "This is why many employers are providing some health services at the work site and are encouraging use of retail clinics for convenience. It is also a reason that employers support advanced medical homes, integrated delivery systems and ACOs [accountable care organizations]. Employers believe that health systems that have incentives to keep people healthy and reduce risks are more likely to have robust 'after-hours' access, not just for emergencies, and multiple ways to have contacts with doctors and advanced practice nurses."

The delivery of health care services exclusively during the typical 9-to-5 weekday window is based in part on the outdated assumption that if we have a chronic illness, we are not working. It is left over from an era when fewer people had chronic conditions, when those who did were unable to work, and when the dominant medical approach was acute care in response to a crisis.

It is now possible for many of us to live long and well with chronic conditions. We are deeply grateful for the advances in medicine and health care that allow us to remain economically productive. But we are also acutely aware that it is not only the tests and drugs that make this possible: It is also when and how we plan for their use with our trusted clinicians.

Our health care should not compromise our job security or ability to work, but rather, should support it.

Make the Most of It

I'm Not Taking That Drug If It Makes Me Itch! More on Medication Adherence

What do people do about uncomfortable, unanticipated side effects of medication?

The answer to this question is often: "Stop taking it."

Our unwillingness to take our medicine as directed is often mistakenly viewed by clinicians and researchers as a sign that we are not "engaged" in our care. Baloney. Many of us would be perfectly happy to take our drugs were it not for those pesky side effects.

This might appear to be a trivial problem unless you are the one with the itch. But given our generally casual approach to medication adherence (estimated to be responsible for more than $290 billion in health care expenses annually), it is worth a closer look at policies, incentives or new delivery system models that might help us out when a new medication makes us itch uncontrollably.[1]

Let's start with how common medication side effects should be handled...

In a *rational world*, I would call my clinician, she returns my call within 12 hours, we talk about it, she suggests cutting the dose or timing it differently or else she prescribes an alternative approach. In an ideal world, this whole interaction takes place within a couple hours online with a member of my care team in my medical home via a patient portal and includes short follow-up email conversations over the coming weeks to monitor both my symptoms and drug side effects.

Is that how it works for you?

That's not how it works for the four people who mentioned this problem to me in the past week. For them, itchiness was the most popular reason to stop taking new prescription medications (followed by wobbly stomach). This is an unscientific sample, to be sure, but the number of complaints in such a short time caught my attention, as did the fact that all of them contacted their clinician to ask whether this reaction was normal and whether they should stop taking the drug. And none of them got a reply within 48 hours. That would be a lot of itching if they had waited for their clinician's OK.

One person reported reading carefully through the package insert, WebMD and the manufacturer's online site to find out about side effects. Itchiness was not one of them, but when he Googled the name of the drug and "itchiness," the search came back with hundreds of reports by people who had the same complaint. Many of them reported that they stopped taking their medication. Note that these people were sufficiently "engaged in their care" to go online to find out if anyone else was scratching.

Is this a trivial problem? Certainly not for any people still taking their medications despite itches and wobbly tummies. Their original complaint remains untreated, plus they have an additional source of discomfort. But is it trivial to clinicians or employers or health plans or anyone concerned about the overall cost of care? Perhaps not.

Drugs that are purchased but not taken are wasted. When we discontinue medication meant to cure disease or manage symptoms, predicted outcomes are less likely to be reached, and this can affect clinician and institutional payment. Employees miss work or are distracted by the original problem or drug side effects.

The size of this problem is unknown, but consider that 60 percent of U.S. adults reported using one or more prescription drugs in 2010.[2] That would be 12 prescriptions per capita.[3] In one year. The number of different medications individuals use means that side effects and drug interactions are more common. What percentage of the nation's $320 billion annual prescription drug expenditures could be reduced — or the effectiveness of that investment improved — by addressing this problem?[4] And just what would it take to address the problem of new side effects, anyway?

Here's what solutions look like from our perspective:

First, I can use Dr. Google. Searching produces a cascade of information, some of it useful (if only to validate my experience), but much of it is biased or inaccurate — as with any Web search, you have to consider the source. Information can reduce uncertainty about the cause but doesn't touch the itching itself. And I risk exacerbating my original complaint by not treating it if I stop taking the drug.

Next, I can head to the pharmacy. Pharmacists are an excellent resource. They can provide accurate information about side effects if I can get one to talk to me. But they don't know my medical history or why my clinician prescribed this medication specifically. I probably will have to provide information about all the other medications I take. And after all this, the pharmacist can suggest alternatives but can't prescribe them.

Another approach is to call that handy medical advice line provided by my health plan. Nurse advice lines present similar challenges to pharmacists, although with less specific drug knowledge.

The best alternative is to talk to my prescribing clinician. He knows me, the history of the problem, my allergies and sensitivities, and he knows why he prescribed this medication as opposed to the generic or a similar one. He could work with me to try different approaches until, together, we find one I can tolerate that will address my original complaint. But this takes time, and my limited sample from last week suggests that many busy clinicians — generalists and specialists alike — just don't have the backup organization to respond to what appears to be a low-level query.

The patient-centered medical home model promotes using a team approach to responding quickly and knowledgeably to such inquiries, supported by a patient portal and secure email communication. But today, most people do not receive primary care in practices organized in this way. Further, a significant percent of prescriptions are written by specialists who lack support and incentives to address this concern.

Why raise this issue?

Because it is a good illustration of how advances in health care simultaneously promise better outcomes for us (so many new drugs that can do so much more!) while demanding more from us (managing side effects, complicated dosing regimens and potential drug interactions!). To realize the potential benefit of all the new prescription medications now available, we need to invest more time and energy into figuring out which ones can do the job, given the trade-offs of effectiveness, side effects, interactions and expense. Obviously, we can't make these calculations alone; we need the ongoing help of our clinicians to do so. But our clinicians have yet to realize the extent to which these additional choices of medications require more and different conversations with us than they are used to or prepared for.

This example also illustrates a slow leak in resources — money and time: ours, our clinicians', our employers' and our hospitals'. This slow leak is one of many that undermine the ability of the nation's investment in health care to reach its potential in improved outcomes.

And for patients and families particularly, it tells a true story about how our efforts to use the tools of health care to live our lives free of suffering are thwarted by a mindset that equates compliance with engagement and inadvertently prevents the kind of collaboration that will give us the best shot at doing so.

Don't Miss the Chance to Engage Us When Introducing Patient-Centered Innovations

Here's the bad news: We will not benefit from the health care services, drugs, tests or procedures available to us unless we pay attention, learn about our choices, interact with our clinicians and follow through on the plans we make together. And that "following through" part? We have to work at doing that every day, whether we feel sick or well, tired or energetic. And if we can't do it, we'd best find a spouse, adult child, parent, friend or someone from a social service agency who can step in to do the things we can't manage.

OK. For some people, this is not bad news. This is how we think it should be: "Nothing about me without me." For others, our personal encounters with tests, treatments and illness have taught us that this is just the way it is.

But for many of us, this news — should we have reason to attend to it — is inconsistent with our idealized vision of health care that, tattered as its image might be, will step in, take over and fix what ails us. Most of us, after all, are mostly well most of the time, and our exposure to health care is minimal.

Efforts to improve the effectiveness of health care and contain its cost have produced a number of innovations designed to help us more easily shoulder some of our new responsibilities for our health and care. But those of us who have yet to recognize the tasks that are now ours often mistake those "patient-centered" innovations as new barriers between us and the help we need.

For example:

- Finding ourselves **cared for by a team** shatters our expectations about having a traditional relationship with our familiar trusted doctor. Without warning, we have lost access to this single authoritative source of care and now must rely on the advice of unfamiliar professionals whose expertise and scope of work we don't understand.

- The promise that our **care will be coordinated** by our primary care clinician is familiar from the last health care reform go-round and is easily misinterpreted that our clinician will act as a gatekeeper (now cleverly disguised) and will restrict the care provided by the specialists we choose.

- Similarly, the convenience of a **patient portal of an electronic health record** that provides secure communication with a team, access to test results and targeted information can be experienced as off-loading responsibility onto patients and creating a barrier to direct communication. This is especially true for those with little computer experience and those who find deciphering medical jargon and monitoring a portal burdensome when ill.

- And I still hear people describe their experience with **shared decision making** as an admission of ignorance by their clinician: ("She's the doctor. Why is she asking me? I don't know what to do. That's why I asked her.") or with concern that this is an attempt by clinicians to shift legal liability to them.

While these innovations are the patient-facing signature of the Patient-Centered Medical Home, primary care practices and clinics all over the country are implementing them as they attempt to meet new expectations about organizational quality and accountability.[1]

Taking some time to introduce these innovations to us within the context of our personal health concerns provides an opportunity for clinicians to discuss patient engagement. That is, how critical it is that each of us participates actively in our care, while at the same time easing fears that a new tool or process signals danger, rejection, laziness or incompetence on our part. So when introducing each of these innovations, how about a conversation that starts: *You know, medicine has advanced a lot in recent years — we can do so much more now about many diseases and conditions. But many of the new approaches require that you really pitch in and work with us to keep you as well and active as possible.*

Within that context, patient-facing innovations make sense: *Our new team approach means that a group of professionals here will...This is who they are and what they do and this is how they will work with and for you.* Or: *In order to make sure you can get questions answered quickly and avoid some of the back-and-forth on the phone and with appointments, we have set up a new patient portal to help us communicate more easily with one another. Do you use a computer?*

Oh, sure. Who has time for this kind of conversation in a busy primary care practice or a clinic? Probably not too many people.

Orienting patients to changes in care delivery "is not always a first step just because it is a matter of how much the practice can effectively manage. In addition, as they start the process, the practice is a little unsure how to communicate it to the patients," reports Diane Cardwell, director of practice transformation at TransforMed, a consulting subsidiary of the American Academy of Family Physicians. Kristen Sanderson, a certified medical assistant at Husson Pediatrics, a Maine Patient-Centered Medical Home pilot site in Bangor, told me that, "As far as letting our patients know about the PCMH: We have a bulletin board in the waiting room explaining what a medical home is and listing the core expectations.[2] We also have signs in the exams room with a brief statement describing a medical home. Currently, we do not do any verbal informing of PCMH." And Leif Solberg and co-authors noted in a recent study in the *Annals of Family Medicine* describing trends in quality as primary care practices transform themselves into patient-centered medical homes: "As we move rapidly as a nation to encourage transformation of traditional primary care practices into patient-centered medical homes, this study adds to the reasons for avoiding unrealistic expectations about the rate of improvement in health or patient experience that will result."[3]

Now, I really do understand that getting the EHR to work properly or trying to redesign care delivery to make use of teams, for example, is a profoundly distracting, time-consuming task. I also understand not wanting to over-promise on specific tools and approaches until they are fully implemented and bug-free.

But I also believe that it is unrealistic to expect that we will easily understand and ably engage in team care, shared decision making, care coordination and patient portals of EHRs. Each of these carries the risk of being misunderstood by us in ways that further disenfranchise our efforts and goodwill unless they are discussed and recognized as the valuable tools they are. The introduction of each innovation offers an opportunity for medical professionals to talk with patients candidly and realistically about the need for us to play an active role in making the best possible use of medicine and the expertise of professionals as we engage in the shared enterprise of keeping us as healthy as possible.

Will We "Just Say No" to Screening Tests?

Will we — you, me, our parents and neighbors — be a significant force in quelling the tide of over-testing for the early detection of disease?

When you have had cancer as many times as I have, you become suspicious that more cancer cells are inside you waiting for some obscure signal to make them leap into action and start multiplying out of control. So you develop a deep attachment to constant testing, despite the high price of time, resources and anxiety, because very occasionally that suspicion is validated by the life-saving (so far for me) early detection of yet another cancer.

I used to think that this sense that I am a mere vessel for latent disease was unique to those of us with serial bad diagnoses. But similar anxious suspicions have seeped into the conversations and consciousness of many healthy people. Anxieties about disease are being nurtured by popular beliefs that our future health is encoded in our DNA. And they are heightened, and in turn calmed, by the decades-long public promotion of the value of screening and early detection tests.

While the science of genomics has far outpaced the public's understanding of the promise, pitfalls and progress of gene-based medicine, the American public has embraced its core idea: Genes are destiny. "She has blue eyes just like her dad." "Alcoholism runs in his family." Every time we are asked for our medical history or complete a genogram, we dredge up the cancers, diabetes, epilepsy and heart disease of our great-grandparents and aunts twice removed. We get the message: "Watch out. What was theirs may be yours." Media reports on the discovery of genes associated with feared diseases, television shows illustrating our ancestors' genetic hold on our skin color, temperament and health, and advertising of new low costs for unlocking future health secrets by getting one's own genome read all contribute to a belief that our bodies contain the seeds of our future diseases.

Many of us welcome the chance to get a mammogram or PSA test or have our doctor check our blood for early signs of diabetes or heart problems. We believe these tests work, and that they prevent illness and death. Our employers encourage testing with messages in our pay envelopes and incentives in our benefits plans. The government and health plans push us to get tests through media campaigns and by making tests free. And it's impossible to quantify the dollar amount that organizations like the American Cancer Society and the American Heart Association have invested over the past three decades in educating, cajoling and scaring us into participating in screening for cancer and heart disease.[1,2] The messages are not nuanced. They are bold, decisive and certain: Your life is in danger if you don't get screened.

In op-ed articles and books, H. Gilbert Welch, M.D., describes how testing-as-prevention results in over-diagnosis, overtreatment and injury, sometimes and for some people.[3,4] He recounts how, as new evidence undermines the claims of the life-saving contributions of screening tests for prostate and ovarian cancer, the enthusiasm for guidelines and of physicians for some screening tests is waning.

Dr. Welch is not alone in alerting the public to change its attitude toward the early detection of disease. Otis Brawley, Shannon Brownlee, Rosemary Gibson, Gary Schwitzer and the Choosing Wisely® campaign of the ABIM Foundation all present vivid cases about the dangers that the public faces from screening.[5-9]

So back to the original question: What is the likelihood that this message will get through to us in sufficient numbers that our actions will affect the demand for screening tests?

Slim, I fear.

Our confidence in the benefits of early detection of disease will not be easily overridden. We hold dear the possibility that whether we are healthy or sick, we can transcend our fate — and our DNA — through a rigorously observed protocol of screening and early detection. Deviating from that protocol is a challenge to our own hopes and to decades of messages from authoritative sources. Further, many of our clinicians share our reluctance to back away from accepted norms about screening. A recent study found that more than half of the primary care physicians polled couldn't untangle personalized risk statistics.[10] They will not be able to recommend taking a more nuanced approach to screening.

Reducing the overuse of screening tests is the responsibility of the scientific, professional and financial stakeholders in health care. Payers can and should refuse to pay for inappropriate tests. They can and should foot the bill for free second opinions.[11] Health plans can and must monitor and provide feedback to individual clinicians. Professional societies can and must ensure that each of their members knows where to find and how to use evidence about how to personalize screening guidelines for individual patients.

Sure, efforts to inform us about the dangers of various screening guidelines will be eagerly adopted by some small percentage of the educated and involved public. But for most of us, the promise we've been sold that we can decipher our genetic fate and then act to alter it by getting screening tests is simply too great to resist.

Check–in-the-Box Medicine: The Blunt Instrument of Policy and Patient Engagement

I sat in a dingy pharmacy near the Seattle airport over the holidays, waiting for an emergency prescription. For over two hours I watched a slow-moving line of people sign a book, pay and receive their prescription(s). The cashier told each customer picking up more than one prescription or a child's prescription to wait on the side. In minutes, the harried, white-haired pharmacist came over to ask each person if he or she was familiar with these medications, describe how to take them, identify the side effects to look out for and demonstrate the size of a teaspoon for pediatric medications. Then he asked the person to repeat back what he or she had heard — this was often done in broken, heavily accented English — and then he patiently went over the parts they didn't understand.

I was impressed. This is what every pharmacy should be like — except, of course, for the dinginess, the creeping line and the fact that it was so crowded I could overhear these conversations. Maybe if we got federal legislation enacted requiring pharmacists to offer counseling with each prescription filled, this kind of attention would be the norm, adherence to medication regimens would improve, and drug-related mishaps would be reduced.[1,2]

Wait a minute. Someone already had that good idea. It was the pharmacists themselves, concerned about the proliferation of pharmaceuticals and the unintended negative consequences it produced, who joined together to back federal legislation that went into effect in 1993.[3] And today when you pick up a prescription at your pharmacy, you sign the book or screen at the register, right? Do you know what you are signing?

Probably not. When you sign, you are affirming that you have been offered personal counseling and are documenting that you declined the pharmacist's guidance about how to take the drug, possible side effects and contraindications.[4]

Pharmacists, who face time constraints, a lack of financial incentives to meet this demand (the law included no provisions for reimbursement for counseling) and a public unaware of its need for counseling and uninterested in hearing more about maintenance drugs, find their original wise intention undermined. The benefit the pharmacists envisioned has been transformed into the time-saving strategy of asking us to check the box and sign the book (or screen pad), which says in tiny print that by signing we are declining assistance. Perhaps there was a time when that offer was given verbally (and in some places, it still is), but the vast majority of us now add our signature, pay the bill and walk away, oblivious to the substantial benefit we have just rejected.

Here's another example of an important interaction that's been reduced to checking the box: advance directives. There is consensus that we are more likely to receive care resonant with our values and preferences when we are unable to make our wishes known if we have completed an advance directive.[5] The Patient Self-Determination Act, passed by Congress in 1991, requires most health institutions to inform all adult patients about their rights to accept or refuse medical or surgical treatment and the right to execute an advance directive.[6] Theoretically this inquiry, delivered at a strategically relevant point for us, should remind us to clarify our wishes with our loved ones, offer guidance about how to do so and then encourage us to distribute the documentation to our clinicians. Notably, similar to pharmacists' medication counseling, patients' discussions about advance directives with health professionals are not reimbursed by public or private insurance.[7]

And so this prompt has become another important interaction between us and our clinicians that has been reduced to a check mark. Try this next time you are asked whether you have an advance directive as part of a hospital intake procedure: Ask a) if someone can give you guidance about creating an advance directive; b) if anyone can provide blank forms for you to complete; and c) whether the facility has the capacity to keep those documents on file so that they can be part of your medical record and thus available if you are admitted through the ER. My bet is you'll come up empty on all counts.

Yet another example of potential check-in-the-box medicine in the making: Advocates for shared decision making, eager to disseminate this approach of collaborative health care, spent considerable energy getting legislation passed in the state of Washington in 2007 that informed consent for treatment should include specific elements of shared decision making.[8] Such a dramatic change in the culture of both patients and professionals is a heavy lift for legislation that includes neither financial incentives nor effective penalties to encourage adoption of new behaviors.

Each of these examples describes a situation for which there is evidence that our actions have a significant impact on how and whether we benefit from specific health care interventions. Not one of these situations can be wholly outsourced to a Web-based tool or pamphlet. The interaction that takes place between us and our health professional is critical to ensure that our needs, preferences, motivations and capacities are addressed in the care we receive going forward. In no instance are provisions made to compensate the health professional for the time and skills required to initiate the discussion. The significance of each of these interactions is such that clinical, patient and scientific advocates have joined together to get legislation and regulation passed and private policies implemented to make sure they take place. And regrettably, the unintended consequence of the policies requiring these interactions is that two of the three have become so routinized that they have been reduced to a check mark.

As a longtime advocate whose aim is to ensure that everyone has the opportunity to talk with their clinician about these and other personal health concerns, I am puzzled by the optimism that drives advocates to believe that the blunt instrument of policy is sufficient to ensure that health professionals will change the way they interact with us about specific concerns. I'm still looking for evidence showing that such policies work: fewer medication injuries, more advance directives, greater satisfaction with care.

Legislation and regulation are seductively simple levers for social change that add legitimacy to the advocates' cause. The unintended consequence — check-in-the-box health care — should make us wary about when and how we use it.

Physician counseling for tobacco use cessation had the potential to become yet another check-in-the-box intervention, but the persistence of advocates, scientists and clinicians and the financial investment of foundations and state and federal governments led to a different outcome.[9] Plan- and institution-level policies requiring clinicians to Ask, Advise, Assist and Arrange for cessation support are supplemented by 1) considerable research support demonstrating the efficacy and value of clinician-initiated counseling for different subgroups; 2) clinician compensation for counseling; 3) insurance coverage for pharmaceutical cessation aids; 4) performance measures of counseling delivery via patient surveys; 5) readily available professional training for a variety of health professionals; 6) free national telephone counseling; and 7) clean indoor air policies and powerful media messages that reinforce quitting.[10-18] Productive interactions between clinicians and patients with regard to tobacco use is, over the past two decades, slowly becoming the norm.[19]

That harried, white-haired pharmacist near the Seattle airport patiently counseling his clients is an exception.[20] What additional measures — what will and what resources — must be taken to ensure that all pharmacists and other health professionals can confidently and gladly engage with us about how to make the best possible use of our health care?

Patient-Centered Care: From Exam Room to Dinner Table

Only one in ten respondents to a national survey could estimate how many calories they should consume in a day.

Seventy-nine percent make few or no attempts to pay attention to the balance between the calories they consume and expend in a day.

These and other piquant findings from the online 2011 Food and Health Survey fielded by the International Food Information Council Foundation (IFIC) struck home last week as I smacked up against my own ignorance about a healthy diet and the difficulty of changing lifelong eating habits.[1]

The confluence of my failure to gain weight after cancer treatment and a blood test suggesting pre-diabetes meant that I have been on an "eat specific types of food every hour and write it down" regimen. And despite a lifetime of recommending that people change their behavior to become healthier, I am frustrated as I try to follow my own advice. I am bewildered about what I'm supposed to eat. Finding it, preparing it and then eating it at the right time requires untold contortions and inconvenience. Writing it all down is tedious. I don't have time for this — I have a job, obligations.

In the midst of my crankiness about this, my admiration is renewed for those who figure out every day how to incorporate into their busy lives the demands of diabetes, allergies and other chronic diseases. How easy it is to underestimate the effort required of people who are ill to become as functional and healthy as they can!

It's ironic that as more is learned about the effect of what we eat on our health, the greater our responsibility has become to make use of that knowledge. But we won't benefit from that knowledge unless we are willing and able to consistently monitor, learn from, tweak and change daily eating habits.

Many of us don't yet realize just how much our health depends on our own actions — food-related and otherwise. And whether we realize it or not, many of us, including me, still struggle to find the skills, time, energy and knowledge to take on these tasks, some of which must be attended to every day for the rest of our lives.

Food plays a central role in many of our lives. We mostly like it. We enjoy food that is familiar; we are concerned about its cost and convenience. It is an integral part of our celebrations and daily routines, our family and social lives.

When a new way of eating is mandated, all of the necessary changes challenge those attributes and experiences. Changes like counting calories, making different food choices, recording what we eat and eating at odd times come at us in unexpected ways, upsetting our assumptions about what is safe to consume and disturbing comfortable habits and expectations.

The extent of our responsibility for changing the way we eat has not escaped the notice of the government, our employers, health plans and providers, however.[2] Their messages to us are an unending stream of general nudges to eat less and differently. In a recent newsletter, the insurer Cigna tells readers to "eat healthy" by consuming a low-calorie diet, advice that will unfortunately baffle 90 percent of the population, according to the IFIC survey cited above. Indeed, the public is only vaguely aware of the government's "Dietary Guidelines for America" and MyPyramid: 68 percent had never heard of them or had heard of them but knew nothing about them.

These public health messages are of little use to those whose food consumption directly increases their risk for disease or to those with chronic conditions that require specific changes in their eating habits. While we are responsible for carrying out those changes, our primary care clinicians also bear the responsibility of informing us about our

Slow Leaks: Missed Opportunities to Encourage Our Engagement in Our Health Care

unique need to change what we eat, educating us about exactly what that means for us, helping us monitor progress and modify our plans, and working with us over time to sustain new habits.[3] That is, if we even have a primary care clinician.

Thus, taking seriously the responsibility for dietary changes is pretty disruptive to our clinicians. Some clinicians have responded to these additional demands on them by sharing some of these tasks with a primary care health care team.[4] Others make referrals to diabetes educators or nutritionists or rely on a care plan, nurse educator and joint use of Web-based education and monitoring — appropriate for people with diabetes but less so for the many other conditions requiring dietary modifications.[5,6] Some just punt, hoping that their advice and a couple of pamphlets will spark our impulse for self-preservation and we will leap into action.

But the responsibilities clinicians bear are modest compared with ours. Making significant dietary changes over time is wildly disruptive to us and those with whom we live. Shopping, preparing, eating and monitoring all have to be done with knowledge, skills, resources and attention. How can our clinicians better help us approach these formidably complex tasks?

Here's an idea. In his vivid talk, Victor Montori, M.D., of the Mayo Clinic talks about what one of his patients must do to address his high blood pressure, his diabetes, his weight and the events in his life that compete for his attention.[7] He describes how guidelines-based care and pay-for-performance incentives inadvertently undermine this patient's willingness to take action. And he proposes that clinicians reorganize the care they deliver to 1) take into account the burden of treatment demands; 2) organize care to minimize disruption; and 3) order treatment priorities from the patient's perspective.

There are few of us whose lives are not so full of responsibilities that we would not benefit from our clinicians' recognition of the level of effort required of us when they recommend complicated changes to our daily routine. At a time when patient-centeredness in health care is a concern of policy makers and clinicians alike, Montori's approach increases the likelihood that we will be able to act on our own behalf. In seeking to mitigate the treatment burden by recognizing both the demands of the treatment and the context in which each patient must meet those demands, this care is consistent with the Institute of Medicine's definition of patient-centered; that is, it is "respectful of and responsive to individual patient preferences, needs and values."[8]

The IFIC survey gives us new opportunity to reflect on just how far we are as a country from knowing how to take on this crucial task — eating better — that gives us the best chance of living long and well. It also shines a clear light on the leap in knowledge, skills and attention that will have to be made by many of us who are diagnosed with nutrition-sensitive conditions as the incidence of pre-diabetes, diabetes and food sensitivities continues to rise.[9]

I'm struggling to make that leap today, and it is not easy. Despite existing efforts to help us change what and how much we eat, we are going to need a little more help.

Introduction

1. Prepared Patient Blog. http://www.cfah.org/blog/

Foreword: Engagement Does Not Mean Compliance

1. Many patients may never fill new prescriptions. Reuters. February 17, 2010. http://www.reuters.com/article/2010/02/17/us-new-prescriptions-study-idUSTRE61G3QX20100217

2. Drug Therapy: Adherence to Medication. NEJM. August 4, 2005. http://www.nejm.org/search?q=353%3A487&

3. Enhancing Prescription Medicine Adherence: A National Action Plan. National Council on Patient Information and Education. August 2007. http://www.talkaboutrx.org/documents/enhancing_prescription_medicine_adherence.pdf

The Rocky Adolescence of Public Reporting on Health Care Quality

1. United States Unemployment Rate. Trading Economics. November 9, 2011. http://www.tradingeconomics.com/united-states/unemployment-rate

2. Income, Poverty, and Health Insurance Coverage in the United States: 2010. U.S. Census Bureau. September 2011. http://www.census.gov/prod/2011pubs/p60-239.pdf

3. Commonwealth Fund: Number of "Underinsured" Adults Has Skyrocketed Since 2003. MyHealthCafe.com. September 12, 2011. http://myhealthcafe.com/commonwealth-fund-number-of-underinsured-adults-has-skyrocketed-since-2003

4. Medical bankruptcy study not so clear-cut. Tampa Bay Times PolitiFact.com. June 11, 2009. http://www.politifact.com/truth-o-meter/statements/2009/jun/11/chris-dodd/medical-bankruptcy-study-not-clear-cut/

5. Public release of performance data in changing the behaviour of healthcare consumers, professionals or organisations. PubMed. November 9, 2011. http://www.ncbi.nlm.nih.gov/pubmed/22071813

6. Public reporting in health care: how do consumer use quality-of-care information? A systematic review. PubMed. January 2009.

http://www.ncbi.nlm.nih.gov/pubmed/19106724

7. Quality and Consumer Decision Making in the Market for Health Insurance and Health Care Services. Medical Care Research and Review. February 2009. http://mcr.sagepub.com/content/66/1_suppl/28S.short

8. Snapshot of People's Engagement in Their Health and Health Care. Center for Advancing Health. May 20, 2010. http://www.cfah.org/engagement/research/snapshot

9. Meaningful Price Information Is Difficult for Consumers to Obtain Prior to Receiving Care. U.S. Government Accountability Office. September 23, 2011. http://www.gao.gov/products/GAO-11-791

10. The State of Health Care Quality. National Committee for Quality Assurance. 2010.http://www.ncqa.org/portals/0/state%20of%20health%20care/2010/sohc%202010%20-%20full2.pdf

11. Getting a Good Report Card: Unintended Consequences of the Public Reporting of Hospital Quality. Agency for Healthcare Research and Quality. November 2006. http://www.webmm.ahrq.gov/case.aspx?caseID=137

12. The Latest EHR Adoption Concerns. EHR Bloggers. April 8, 2011. http://www.practicefusion.com/ehrbloggers/2011/04/latest-ehr-adoption-concerns.html

13. Evidence That Consumers Are Skeptical About Evidence-Based Health Care. Health Affairs. June 2010. http://content.healthaffairs.org/content/early/2010/06/03/hlthaff.2009.0296.abstract

14. The High Concentration of U.S. Health Care Expenditures. Agency for Healthcare Research and Quality. June 2006. http://www.ahrq.gov/research/ria19/expendria.htm

15. Understanding U.S. Health Care Spending. National Institute for Health Care Management. July 2011. http://nihcm.org/images/stories/NIHCM-CostBrief-Email.pdf

16. Higher Copayments and Deductibles Delay Medical Care, A Common Problem for Americans. Managed Care. January 2010. http://www.managedcaremag.com/archives/1001/1001.downstream.html

17. Who Doesn't Gather Health Information Online? Pew Research Center. October 18, 2011. http://pewinternet.org/Commentary/2011/

October/Who-Doesnt-Gather-Health-Information-Online.aspx

What Must We Know About What Our Doctors Know

1. The Problem of Fragmentation and the Need for Integrative Solutions. Annals of Family Medicine. March 1, 2009. http://www.annfammed. org/content/7/2/100.full

2. National Priorities Partnership and the National Quality Strategy (NQS). National Quality Forum. September 11, 2011. http://www. qualityforum.org/Setting_Priorities/NPP/Input_into_the_National_ Quality_Strategy.aspx

3. Improving the Quality of Transitional Care for Persons with Complex Care Needs. Journal of the American Geriatrics Society. 2003. http://www.caretransitions.org/definitions.asp

4. Patient-Centered Primary Care Collaborative. http://www.pcpcc.net/

5. The Family Experience with Primary Care Physicians and Staff. National Alliance on Mental Illness. May 2011. http://www.nami. org/template.cfm?template=/contentmanagement/contentdisplay. cfm&contentid=120671

6. National Alliance on Mental Illness. http://www.nami.org/

7. Crossing the Quality Chasm: A New Health System for the 21st Century. Institute of Medicine. March 1, 2001. http://www.iom.edu/ Reports/2001/Crossing-the-Quality-Chasm-A-New-Health-System- for-the-21st-Century.aspx

Semper Paratus: Our Decisions About Emergency Care

1. What is Urgent Care? MedExpress. http://medexpress.com/why- medexpress/what-is-urgent-care.aspx

2. Disputes over coverage of emergency department services: A study of two health maintenance organizations. Annals of Emergency Medicine. February 2004. http://www.annemergmed.com/article/S0196-0644(03)00637-1/ abstract

3. Emergency Room - Typical Average Cost of Hospital ED Visit. Consumer Health Ratings.com. http://www.consumerhealthratings. com/index.php?action=showSubCats&cat_id=274

4. National Hospital Ambulatory Medical Care Survey: 2006 Emergency Department Summary. National Health Statistics Reports. August 6,

2008. http://www.cdc.gov/nchs/data/nhsr/nhsr007.pdf

5. Healthwise Handbook. Healthwise. http://www.healthwise.org/
    Questions.aspx

6. Is it an Emergency? American College of Emergency Physicians.
    http://www.emergencycareforyou.org/EmergencyManual/
    IsItAnEmergency/Default.aspx

7. When to Go to the Emergency Room. Healthywomen. May 6, 2010.
    http://www.healthywomen.org/content/blog-entry/when-go-
    emergency-room

8. Emergency Department Visits. CDC. http://www.cdc.gov/nchs/
    fastats/ervisits.htm

9. Emergency Department Overuse. Providing the Wrong Care at the
    Wrong Time. New England Healthcare Institute. http://bit.ly/12Bbaji

10. Seeking care for nonurgent medical conditions in the emergency
    department: Through the eyes of the patient. Journal of Emergency
    Nursing. December 2000. http://www.ncbi.nlm.nih.gov/
    pubmed/11106453

11. A Dollars and Sense Strategy to Reducing Frequent Use of Hospital
    Services. The California Endowment and the California HealthCare
    Foundation. October 2008. http://documents.csh.org/documents/
    fui/FUHSISummaryReportFINAL.pdf

12. Emergency Room Wait Times Up, But So Is Patient Satisfaction.
    MedPage Today. June 22, 2009. http://www.medpagetoday.com/
    EmergencyMedicine/EmergencyMedicine/14820

13. Emergency Room - Typical Average Cost of Hospital ED Visit.
    Consumer Health Ratings.com. http://www.consumerhealthratings.
    com/index.php?action=showSubCats&cat_id=274

14. Creating a Patient Guide for a "Medical Home" Physician Practice.
    The Center for Advancing Health. 2009. http://www.cfah.org/file/
    CFAH_PACT_Guide_Medical_Home.pdf

Dicker With Your Doc? Not So Fast...

1. How to Haggle With Your Doctor. The New York Times. January 7,
    2011.
    http://well.blogs.nytimes.com/2011/01/07/how-to-haggle-with-
    your-doctor/

2. How to Cut Your Doctor Bill. Forbes.com. July 15, 2009. http://www.forbes.com/fdc/welcome_mjx.shtml

3. Save Big: Negotiate With Your Doctor. ABC News. June 14, 2010. http://abcnews.go.com/Business/save-big-negotiate-doctor/story?id=10888443

4. Contact Your Doctor, Request and Document the Price. Healthcare Blue Book. http://healthcarebluebook.com/page_ContactDoctor.aspx

5. Health Care: The Disquieting Truth. The New York Review of Books. September 30, 2010. http://www.nybooks.com/articles/archives/2010/sep/30/health-care-disquieting-truth/?pagination=false&printpage=true

6. Evidence That Consumers Are Skeptical About Evidence-Based Health Care. Health Affairs. July 2010. http://content.healthaffairs.org/content/29/7/1400.abstract

7. Healthcare Organizations Link Physician Pay to Performance. News-Medical.Net. September 17, 2010. http://www.news-medical.net/news/20100917/Healthcare-organizations-link-physician-pay-to-performance.aspx

8. Drug Protocol Management: Step Therapy. Express Scripts. 2002. https://member.express-scripts.com/images/pdf/step_therapy.pdf

Are Patient Navigators Necessary or Just Nice?

1. Snapshot of People's Engagement in Their Health and Health Care. Center for Advancing Health. May 20, 2010. http://www.cfah.org/engagement/research/snapshot

2. The Coming Age of the Patient Navigator Media Health Leaders. Media Health Leaders. April 26, 2011. http://www.healthleadersmedia.com/print/MAG-264896/The-Coming-Age-of-the-Patient-Navigator

3. Harold P. Freeman Patient Navigation Institute. http://www.hpfreemanpni.org/about-us/

4. A Model Patient Navigation Program. Oncology Issues. September/October 2004. http://accc-cancer.org/oncology_issues/articles/sepoc04/freeman.pdf

5. Breast Patient Navigator Certification Program. National Consortium of Breast Centers. http://www.bpnc.org/about-bpnc.cfm

6. Right This Way: Patient Navigators Provide Guidance. DukeHealth. org. http://www.dukehealth.org/health_library/health_articles/right-this-way

7. Colonoscopy Patient Navigator Program Orientation Manual. NYC Health. 2007. http://www.nyc.gov/html/doh/downloads/pdf/cancer/orientation.pdf

8. Women At Risk. New York-Presbyterian. http://nyp.org/services/war/

9. Elder Patient Navigator Program 2.0. University of Massachusetts Medical School. http://www.pogoe.org/productid/20768

10. Patients Get Personalized Pampering at Stanford Cancer Center. Stanford Medicine. http://cancer.stanford.edu/features/patient_care_news/personalized_care.html

11. Tools for Community Cancer Centers. Association of Community Cancer Centers. http://www.accc-cancer.org/education/patientnavigation-PNT2009-toc.asp

12. Clinical Navigator Job Description. Fox Chase Virtua Health Cancer Program. 2009. http://accc-cancer.org/education/pdf/PNTOOLS2009/Clinical-Navigator.pdf

13. Oncology Nursing Society, the Association of Oncology Social Work, and the National Association of Social Workers Joint Position on the Role of Oncology Nursing and Oncology Social Work in Patient Navigation. http://www.ons.org/Publications/Positions/Navigation

14. Harold P. Freeman Patient Navigation Institute. http://www.hpfreemanpni.org/the-program/

15. Colorado Patient Navigator Training. http://patientnavigatortraining.org/website/about.htm

16. Cancer Patient Navigation: Where Do We Go From Here? Oncology Issues. May/June 2010. http://accc-cancer.org/oncology_issues/articles/mayjune10/MJ10-VarnerMurph.pdf

17. Patient Navigation: A Call to Action. National Association of Social Workers. 2007. http://www.thefreelibrary.com/Patient+navigation%3a+a+call+to+action.-a0161396390

18. 'Patient Navigator' Serves As Guide On Cancer Journey. American Cancer Society. January 25, 2008. http://www.cancer.org/cancer/news/features/patient-navigator-serves-as-guide-on-cancer-journey

Are We All Ready for Do-It-Yourself Health Care?

1. The Net Delusion: The Dark Side of Internet Freedom. Amazon. http://www.amazon.com/s/ref=nb_sb_noss?url=search-alias%3Dstripbooks&field-keywords=Evgeny+Mozorov%3BNet+Delusion&x=0&y=0

2. Wellness, Cost-Cutting Main Themes at Health 2.0 Spring Event. iHealthBeat. March 28, 2011. http://www.ihealthbeat.org/features/2011/wellness-cost-cutting-main-themes-at-health-2-0-spring-event.aspx

3. Digital Divide Threatens Health Care. Kaiser Health News. January 11, 2011. http://www.kaiserhealthnews.org/Stories/2011/January/11/health-digital-divide-cpi.aspx

4. The Digital Divide in Adoption and Use of a Personal Health Record. Archives of Internal Medicine. March 2011. http://archinte.jamanetwork.com/article.aspx?articleid=226918

5. Snapshot of People's Engagement in Their Health Care. Center for Advancing Health. May 20, 2010. http://www.cfah.org/engagement/research/snapshot

6. Prescription for Trouble: Medicare Part D and Patterns of Computer and Internet Access Among the Elderly. Journal of Aging and Social Policy. March 30, 2009. http://www.tandfonline.com/doi/abs/10.1080/08959420902732514

7. Purchasing Health Insurance Online: Full Report. California HealthCare Foundation. December 2002. https://www.ehealthinsurance.com/content/expertcenterNew/OnlineInsuranceFullReport.pdf

8. Attributes of Interactive Online Health Information Systems. Journal of Medical Internet Research. 2005. http://www.jmir.org/2005/3/e33/

9. Electronic Health Records and Meaningful Use. The Office of the National Coordinator for Health Information Technology. February 9, 2011.
http://healthit.hhs.gov/portal/server.pt?open=512&objID=2996&mode=2

Why Can I Only Get Health Care from 9—5, M—F ?

1. Financial and Health Burdens of Chronic Conditions Grow. Center for

Studying Health System Change. April 2009. http://www.hschange.com/CONTENT/1049/

2. The Chronic Care Model. The Robert Wood Johnson Foundation. http://www.improvingchroniccare.org/index.php?p=the_chronic_care_model&s=2

3. Federally Qualified Health Centers A Medical Home Model That Works! New Jersey Primary Care Association. 2010. http://www.njpca.org/Medical%20Home%20Document.pdf

4. The Most Commonsensical And Hopeless Reform Idea Ever. Kaiser Health News. June 28, 2011. http://www.kaiserhealthnews.org/Columns/2011/June/062811millenson.aspx

5. Paid Sick Days Campaign. National Partnership for Women and Families. http://www.nationalpartnership.org/site/PageServer?pagename=issues_campaigns_paidsickdays

I'm Not Taking That Drug If It Makes Me Itch! More on Medication Adherence

1. NEHI Research Shows Patient Medication Nonadherence Costs Health Care System $290 Billion Annually. New England Healthcare Institute. August 11, 2009. http://www.nehi.net/news/press_releases/110/nehi_research_shows_patient_medication_nonadherence_costs_health_care_system_290_billion

2. Prescription Drug Accessibility and Affordability in the United States and Abroad. The Commonwealth Fund. June 2010. http://www.commonwealthfund.org/~/media/Files/Publications/Issue%20Brief/2010/Jun/1408_Morgan_Prescription_drug_accessibility_US_intl_ib.pdf

3. United States: Prescription Drugs. The Henry J. Kaiser Family Foundation. http://www.statehealthfacts.org/profileind.jsp?sub=66&rgn=1&cat=5

4. Prescription Drug Spending Was Flat in 2011. USA TODAY. April 4, 2012. http://www.usatoday.com/money/industries/health/drugs/story/2012-04-04/prescription-drug-spending-2011/54000818/1

Don't Miss the Chance to Engage Us When Introducing Patient-Centered Innovations

1. Patient-Centered Primary Care Collaborative. http://www.pcpcc.net/about/medical-home

2. Maine Patient-Centered Medical Home Pilot. Patient-Centered Primary Care Collaborative. http://www.mainequalitycounts.org/page/896-659/patient-centered-medical-home

3. Trends in Quality During Medical Home Transformation. Annals of Family Medicine. November/December2011. http://www.annfammed.org/content/9/6/515.full.pdf+html

Will We "Just Say No" to Screening Tests?

1. Cancer Facts and Figures. American Cancer Society. 2011.http://www.cancer.org/acs/groups/content/@epidemiologysurveilance/documents/document/acspc-029771.pdf

2. Know Your Risks! American Heart Association. http://www.goredforwomen.org/understand_your_risks.aspx

3. If You Feel O.K., Maybe You Are O.K. The New York Times. February 27, 2012. http://www.nytimes.com/2012/02/28/opinion/overdiagnosis-as-a-flaw-in-health-care.html?_r=3

4. Should I Be tested for Cancer? University of California Press. March 2006. http://www.ucpress.edu/book.php?isbn=9780520248366

5. Doctor Exposes the Dangers of Overtreatment. USA TODAY. January 31, 2012. http://www.usatoday.com/news/health/story/health/story/2012-01-30/Doctor-exposes-the-dangers-of-overtreatment/52893278/1

6. Overtreated. http://www.youtube.com/watch?v=gEMPPIOIuIE

7. The Author Speaks: Overtested, Overmedicated, and Overtreated. AARP. April 8, 2010. http://www.aarp.org/health/longevity/info-04-2010/the_author_speaks_overtested_overmedicated_and_overtreated.html

8. HealthNewsReview.org. http://www.healthnewsreview.org/category/screening/

9. Choosing Wisely. American Board of Internal Medicine Foundation. http://www.abimfoundation.org/Initiatives/Choosing-Wisely.aspx

10. Do Physicians Understand Cancer Screening Statistics? A National Survey of Primary Care Physicians in the United States. Annals of Internal Medicine. March 6, 2012. http://annals.org/article.aspx?volume=156&issue=5&page=340

11. Take Patients Away from the Overtreaters. The Treatment Trap.

February 14, 2012. http://www.treatmenttrap.org/

Check-in-the-Box Medicine: The Blunt Instrument of Policy and Patient Engagement

1. Pharmacist Communication Shown to Increase Medication Adherence and Reduce Errors. National Association of Boards of Pharmacy. April 30, 2010. http://www.nabp.net/news/pharmacist-communication-shown-to-increase-medication-adherence-and-reduce-errors/

2. Quantifying Adverse Drug Events: Med Mishaps Send Millions Back for Care. amednews.com. June 13, 2011. http://www.ama-assn.org/amednews/2011/06/13/prl20613.htm

3. OBRA '90 at Sweet Sixteen: A Retrospective Review. U.S. Pharmacist. March 20, 2008. http://www.uspharmacist.com/content/d/featured_articles/c/10126/

4. OBRA '90 Is a Law Passed by the? Yahoo! Answers. 2007. http://answers.yahoo.com/question/index?qid=20080130074133AANQXdb

5. Living Wills and Advance Directives for Medical Decisions. Mayo Clnic. http://www.mayoclinic.com/health/living-wills/HA00014

6. Health Care Advance Directives. American Bar Association. http://www.americanbar.org/groups/public_education/resources/law_issues_for_consumers/patient_self_determination_act.html

7. U.S. Alters Rule on Paying for End-of-Life Planning. The New York Times. January 4, 2011. http://www.nytimes.com/2011/01/05/health/policy/05health.html?_r=1

8. Shared Decision Making Policy. Informed Medical Decisions Foundation. http://informedmedicaldecisions.org/shared-decision-making-policy/

9. State Tobacco Data and Resources L-M. National Association of Local Boards of Health. January 4, 2012. http://www.nalboh.org/State%20Tobacco%20Pages/ST_Tobacco_L_M.htm

10. Effectiveness of Smoking Cessation Therapies: a Systematic Review and Meta-Analysis. BMC Public Health. December 11, 2006. http://www.biomedcentral.com/1471-2458/6/300

11. Interventions to Promote Smoking Cessation in the Medicare Population. RAND Health. 2003. http://www.rand.org/content/dam/

rand/pubs/reprints/2007/RAND_RP1224.sum.pdf

12. Smoking Cessation. Medicare.gov. http://www.medicare.gov/
navigation/manage-your-health/preventive-services/smoking-
cessation.aspx

13. Reimbursement for Smoking Cessation: A Healthcare Practitioner's
Guide. Professional Assisted Cessation Therapy. 2002. http://
www.endsmoking.org/resources/reimbursementguide/pdf/
reimbursementguide-2nd-edition.pdf

14. Scoring Documentation for Consumer Reporting Office of Patient
Advocate HMO CAHPS Reporting Year 2010. Pacific Business Group
on Health. January, 2011. http://reportcard.opa.ca.gov/rc2011/pdfs/
Scoring%20Documentation_HMO%20CAHPS_Consumer%20
Reporting_January%202011.pdf

15. Training in Tobacco Cessation Counseling for Medical, Nursing,
Dentistry and Pharmacy Students: Environmental Scan and
Recommendations. Canadian PUblic Health Association. December
29, 2006. http://www.cpha.ca/uploads/progs/substance/tobacco/
chpscstudyfinal.pdf

16. North American Quitline Consortium. http://www.naquitline.org/

17. List of Smoking Bans in the United States. Wikipedia. http://
en.wikipedia.org/wiki/List_of_smoking_bans_in_the_United_States

18. American Legacy Foundation - Truth Campaign. Social Marketing
Wiki. http://www.legacyforhealth.org/what-we-do/national-
education-campaigns/keeping-young-people-from-using-tobacco

19. Smoking Cessation Treatment by Primary Care Physicians: An Update
and Call for Training. American Journal of Preventive Medicine. July
25, 2006.
http://www.ajpmonline.org/article/S0749-3797(06)00174-7/
abstract

20. A Father's Lessons. Dallas Blog. June 14, 2011. http://www.dallasblog.
com/201106141008166/john-browning-s-legally-speaking/a-father-
s-lessons.html

Patient-Centered Care: From Exam Room to Dinner Table

1. 2011 Food & Health Survey. International Food Information Council
Foundation. May 5, 2011. http://bit.ly/mARYVt

2. Excerpts from the Future of Food conference. The Washington

Post. May 10, 2011. http://www.washingtonpost.com/lifestyle/
food/editors-note-on-the-future-of-food-conference/2011/05/09/
AFEmnojG_story.html

3.   Doctors Don't Discuss Weight Loss With Patients. ACP Internist. May
     2, 2011. http://blog.acpinternist.org/2011/05/doctors-dont-discuss-
     weight-loss-with.html

4.   Medical Home and Diabetes Care. Patient-Centered Primary Care
     Collaborative. http://www.pcpcc.net/guide/practices-spotlight

5.   The Diabetes Care Management Program. Kaiser Permanente.
     2007. http://mydoctor.kaiserpermanente.org/ncal/Images/care_
     management_tcm28-15453.pdf

6.   Managing Diabetes for a Healthy and Active Life. http://mydoctor.
     kaiserpermanente.org/ncal/Images/care_management_tcm28-
     15453.pdf

7.   Minimally Disruptive Medicine - Victor Montori, M.D. You Tube.
     September 9, 2010. http://www.youtube.com/watch?v=flcRKdoaiVk

8.   Crossing the Quality Chasm: A New Health System for the 21st
     Century. Institute of Medicine. March 2001. http://bit.ly/hShr5O

9.   National Diabetes Fact Sheet, 2011. CDC. 2011.
     http://www.cdc.gov/diabetes/pubs/pdf/ndfs_2011.pdf

Jessie Gruman

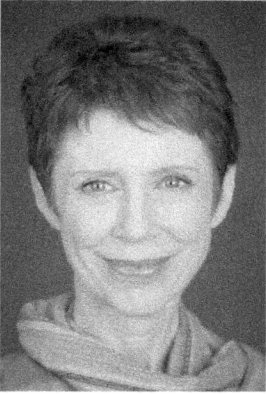

Jessie Gruman is president and founder of the Center for Advancing Health, a nonpartisan, Washington-based policy institute which, since 1992, has been supported by foundations and individuals to work on people's engagement in their health care from the patient perspective. Dr. Gruman draws on her own experience of treatment for four cancer diagnoses, interviews with patients and caregivers, surveys and peer-reviewed research as the basis of her work to describe and advocate for policies and practices to overcome the challenges people face in finding good care and getting the most from it.

Dr. Gruman has worked on this same set of concerns in the private sector (AT&T), the public sector (National Cancer Institute) and the voluntary health sector (American Cancer Society). She holds a B.A. from Vassar College and a Ph.D. in Social Psychology from Columbia University and is a Professorial Lecturer in the School of Public Health and Health Services at the George Washington University. She currently serves on the boards of the Center for Medical Technology Policy, VillageCare in New York City and the Sallan Foundation.

Dr. Gruman has received honorary doctorates from Brown University, Carnegie Mellon University, Clark University, Georgetown University, New York University, Northeastern University, Salve Regina University, Syracuse University and Tulane University, and the Presidential Medal of the George Washington University. She was honored by Research!America for her leadership in advocacy for health research, is a fellow of the Society for Behavioral Medicine and the New York Academy of Medicine and a member of the American Academy of Arts and Sciences and the Council on Foreign Relations.

Dr. Gruman is the author of AfterShock: What to Do When the Doctor Gives You — or Someone You Love — a Devastating Diagnosis (Walker Publishing, second edition, 2010); The Experience of the American Patient: Risk, Trust and Choice (Health Behavior Media, 2009); Behavior Matters (Health Behavior Media, 2008) as well as scientific papers, opinion essays and articles. She blogs regularly on the Prepared Patient Blog at cfah.org/blog and tweets daily @jessiegruman.

www.ingramcontent.com/pod-product-compliance
Lightning Source LLC
Chambersburg PA
CBHW050604280326
41933CB00011B/1980